Break Those Chains.

Preface

- *Those who are serious and are not merely looking for comfort and stupid gains will find great value in those conversations with us.*

- *This book is **NOT** a collection of techniques and methods on how to quit the addiction to pornography and masturbation.*

- *The information given in this compilation of conversations with us must be seen as the starting point of a personal and independent research.*

- *If you have severe addiction or sexual behavior disorder, you must consult a professional of the domain and not rely on this guide or anything said inside of it as a therapy.*

- *We have designed the order of the book in a progressive journey of self-exploration which has been proven to be effective for those who are looking for an alternative way to deal with the addiction to pornography and masturbation.*

Contents

InnerNoPmo

An Endless Suffering

"My face in the mirror..."

It's 2 in the morning...

Suddenly, you wake up with that pressing and burning excitement...

A tingling sensation in your belly, in your feet; your heart is beating very fast spreading the sensation all across your body and your breath accelerates.

You feel blood rushing everywhere in your body...

An erection... A strong one!

-**"Oh no! Not again..."** You say to yourself.

The tension is building up...

It is almost insupportable, unbearable.

-**"*I will not... I will not fail this time...*"** You say, trying to hold on to the last piece of determination you can find.

But you know it's too late...

It is already there!

No matter how much you fight and resist, it seems to be stronger than you, unstoppable, uncontrollable. You can't prevent it from following its course.

The urge is there and you can't help but freak out because you know, from past experiences, what will happen. You know it won't leave you until it gets what it wants.

You don't know what to do...

It controls you.

It has already taken full control of the body like a parasite contaminating everything it touches.

A video... It wants you to open your phone...

-**"*Noo... I... won't...*"** You keep trying.

*"**Come on!** It whispers to your ears, **you remember that video you saw the other day?**"*

It is gaining control of your mind...

-*"**Noo... I... don't wa...**"*

-*"**SHUT UP AND DO IT!**"*

It becomes violent...

You want to cry but your sadness is not its problem, it just wants what it wants regardless of how you feel.

And even worse than that, your resistance strengthens it, gives it more power. The more you fight back, the more insupportable it becomes.

You don't know what to do...

You are alone and no one can help you.

-*"**Perhaps It will go away if I do what it wants**"* You say to yourself.

-*"**But I will lose my 15 days streak and my gains...**"*

-**"You can always start again"** It says to you, while making you imagine the pleasure you will get if you let go.

… Which you do…

Congratulations, you have just <u>RELAPSED</u>!

Does that sound like you?

You see, you have tried so many times and failed so many times to quit and eliminate this secret habit you carry. It is ruining your life.

You have listened to all kind of theories, all kind of "gurus", and all kind of specialists who say they know how to help you. And they have been promising you great outcomes, great transformation and another type of life.

But none of those things really helped. Did they? None of them have shown you any valuable way to deal with this problem you are caught in.

It is making a misery out of your life and you are tired of trying and failing all the time!

Even though you keep relapsing, you get no real pleasure in it because you feel used, controlled and powerless. You no longer have that excitement and sense of enjoyment you had the very first time you did it, there is nothing new, the same old action and the same old feeling.

This burning desire and that frustration are there, present all the time in the back of your soul. It is there when you are by yourself in your room; it is there when you talk with people and they can feel it too; it is there when you open your browser; it is there when you're scrolling in your social media feed and see that sexy post.

It is there and ready to take over at any moment.

And despite all of the methods, all of the theories, all the logics, all the warnings of doctors and religious leaders, you cannot stop it from showing its ugly head.

So, you suffer in silence.

There is nobody to whom you can reach and talk openly about it.

A massive and burdensome feeling of shame ties both your mouth and your heart. And this feeling manifests itself as depression and a sentiment of loneliness, of not being understood.

You hide it.

You hide it from your parents, your family, your friends, your classmates, your roommates, from everyone you know. You even lie sometimes when they ask you about it...

But no matter how good you are in dissimulating it to your surroundings; you can never lie to yourself.

Your life is reduced to a fight you seem to never win. It is consuming everything you are; it affects your mind, your body, your energy, your relationships, your focus, your humanity, every piece of you.

So, with a heart filled with despair, you ask yourself:

"What should I do with that thing?"

"How can I deal with it?"

Is there really a way to quit it definitively?

Am I doomed with that misery forever?"

If you felt that those words were describing your reality and what you are facing on a daily basis, your daily struggle, then this book is definitively for you.

This document you hold in your hands is a mirror which allows you to look at the addiction right in the eyes, exactly as it is, without shame or blame, without guilt, which means without any form of distortion.

We do not pretend in any way to be experts or some kind of specialists or some therapists, offering methods and successful outcomes, but we invite you to explore with us, together, as brothers in the same situation, with the same concern, the same drive, we invite you to question some basic (and yet very important) unconscious beliefs you hold about this condition and to understand the whole meaning and expression of the addiction to pornography and masturbation.

That's the call.

And it is a challenge!

Yes, we challenge you, in our interaction, to find out for yourself, not because someone else tells you, but to discover for yourself, whether or not there is a real way out of that addiction.

And also, think about this...

Wouldn't it be great and noble to leave a valuable, a powerful and helpful discovery in the domain to future generations, your children, who will for sure have that same problem with pornography and masturbation, as we do today?

If you feel that deep concern within your heart, then this book is exactly the tool you were looking for.

Our Community

"Same blood, same struggle..."

Maybe you find yourself asking who we are and how come we know you so well. At least, that part of you we have described in the first pages.

Who are those guys?

Let us introduce ourselves.

We are InnerNoPmo.

InnerNoPmo is a recovery community created by men who have struggled with the addiction to masturbation and pornography.

If you are reading our guide, chances are you are a prey and victim of the addiction; and you are frustrated for seeing no results after applying promising methods, tired of counting days and failing to complete the streaks.

We know what you are going through because we too have followed all the methods you can think of: Intense Sports, Cold Showers, Pushups in the middle of the night, Meditation, Affirmations, Specific Therapies, Pills, and so on...

But none of them have been able to bring that definitive transformation we were looking for.

None. Of. Them.

Out of deception and confusion, we have decided from now on to follow nobody and to take care of the problem ourselves, to take our total responsibility for it.

All the advises, all the methods, all the gurus, all the YouTube videos, all the articles, all the streaks, all the promises and all that culture built on the internet around how to quit porn and masturbation, we have rejected it all!

We have chosen to stand on our own and to do the work ourselves!

And, what happened next was absolutely incredible...

We have then dedicated the following year studying and observing everything we possibly could about the addiction, from our own standpoint.

From the urges to that painful feeling we all experience after a relapse; from the tendency to watch porn to the tendency to judge and blame oneself after orgasm, after a relapse.

We have covered it all, inquiring, digging carefully into the core of what masturbation really is and why we are so attached to it.

Studying and observing ourselves has literally turned into a passion!

We were so fascinated by what we were discovering about the addiction and most important about ourselves.

And while we were exploring ourselves in relation to the habit and trying to understand the whole thing, we have noticed something really magical...

We have noticed the urges starting to show themselves less frequently!

It was as if the addiction has lost its power or as if the mind was no longer interested in following that pattern it has been conditioned to for so many years.

The urges became less and less violent, less and less important.

A transformation has occurred!

We were free from the grip of our tyrant!

And it has happened without us having to fight or to resist ourselves. Without having to follow any kind of methods.

You could say that it has happened in a natural way.

As a natural consequence of getting a full insight into what was keeping us attached to pornography and masturbation, and as a consequence of having discovered the hidden source where the urges were coming from and what their purpose was.

And, that somewhat magical change that occurred in our minds and even our bodies kept mysteriously growing, expanding itself in other aspects of our lives.

Not only has it freed us from the addiction, but it has also brought a sense of maturity, of responsibility, of peace, of order, of clarity in our judgement, a sense of certain grasp of our lives, a sense of self-confidence, of fearlessness, a sense of wonder, of beauty and of pleasantness in everything that we touch.

It is so strange and painfully difficult to describe.

It was as if something inside of each one of us has opened up, something has grown or matured.

And, having come upon this mysterious and yet magnificent "Thing", automatically sets us on this great mission: To share it with those who are suffering with that same problem we had.

For that purpose, we consider any man struggling with the pain, the deception and the confusion produced by the addiction to masturbation, and seriously looking for a change, as our brother.

No matter where he lives, which race he belongs to or the culture he identifies himself with.

It doesn't even matter how old he is and how long he has been suffering in that condition.

He is our brother.

We feel this strong connection with him because we have the same background, which is the addiction. We have the same blood, which is the sincere desire to bring a real transformation.

By sharing that same drive, that same concern. It unites us, doesn't it?

That's why we can understand each other.

So, we are not at all different and our connection, through this work, is the relationship of brothers walking together in the same direction.

Adding to that the fact that if we unite ourselves by discovering, learning, by exploring and observing together, we can go very far and you can find out how to deal with that plague in your life and perhaps leave something behind for future generations, your sons.

We are together in that exploration.

But you see brother, for us to have a meaningful and helpful communication, for us to take that journey together, we first have to get certain things right...

Because our walk together demands *seriousness, responsibility* and the *drive to inquire.*

And those three basic requirements can be found in one single attitude:

Humility!

Only with that kind of attitude can we communicate and build something together, isn't it?

If you confine yourself in some fixed ideas and point of views, we can never have a good and productive communication.

But if we do share the same reality and the same passion then we can walk together in the park and converse on our problems to find a solution, as true friends do, as brothers do.

- We are being humble when we admit to ourselves the simple fact that we don't know how to deal with the addiction and the other simple fact that the things we have been holding as truth about it up until now haven't really helped.

- We are being humble when we stop running after promises, after gains and what we imagine the transformation to be, when we stop the childish tendency to expect superficial results. Which is, by the way, is what we mean by seriousness.

- We are being humble when we sincerely want to discover why we are the way we are, when we honestly want to understand our addiction through self-inquiry.

Therefore dear brother, humility is our greatest tool. It is what will keep the conversation flowing in the right direction for <u>both</u> of us.

Yes, for both of us, because we also, we will try to flow with humility by not trying to convince you of anything, not trying to impose any of our ideas on you and by respecting your freedom to inquiry and to discover for yourself.

Can we do that? It's our strong brotherly agreement.

Now, some of the points we will touch in this book will make you feel uncomfortable, some will turn you upside down, some will shake you up, some will be difficult to grasp on the first try, some will create disturbance in the way you perceive yourself and the addiction.

But don't be afraid, that's normal, keep moving, we are going together and we will let nothing stop us
(It's a real challenge, always remember that).

For that purpose, we will go as simple and as direct as we can, carefully, breaking it down into simple terms, so that none of our brothers is left behind, gently, with calm, exploring the whole problem in a meaningful and truthful manner.

And, above all, please remember that this work is entirely about <u>YOU</u>, which means it should be fun and exciting every step of the way!

The Traditional Approach

"A leak in the system..."

Here we are with our addiction to masturbation and watching pornography. And here we are with our shame and our guilt.

Here you are with the urges coming and fulfilling themselves against your will. Here you are like a slave.

And, since the day you have realized your addiction to PMO, you have wanted the situation to change.

So, with that aspiration in your heart, you have followed the trend.

You do what everyone else on the "journey" of NOT- FAPPING is doing: You fight...

You follow methods, cold showers, sport, meditation and all the ways the "gurus" offer. You resist, you blame yourself and try to control the urges.

And the longer you keep that fight going, the harder it becomes. The longer your streak, the prouder you feel...

...Until you relapse.

And when this happens, when you "*lose*" your streak, the whole world collapses; the entire universe feels bitter and cruel.

Your self-esteem drops, depression kicks in, you feel ugly, dirty and worthless.

And, oh boy! This is not at all a good time!

This is what we call the **"Traditional Approach"** in our community, the way of the fighter.

You see, this way of dealing with PMO (Pornography, Masturbation and Orgasm) has been around for a very long time and we have all accepted it as the only approach capable of bringing a transformation in our lives.

But when you look at what is actually going on in the culture created around that approach, very few have been able to free themselves using this traditional approach.

As a matter fact, if we are being brutally honest with ourselves, we must admit that most of us can't even hold more than one week without relapsing.

This, brother, is an eye-opening indication of a certain limitation of this system. Isn't it?

Either that system doesn't match the problem we are facing or the vast majority of us are not fit for the system. Either way, some questions must be asked!

Some serious questions because we are talking about millions of guys around the world struggling, fighting against PMO, following the traditional approach, and trusting it, consciously or unconsciously, to bring a change, leaning on it to free them.

But it is not working...

All of us, we are still suffering the relapses and the pain that goes with them.

So, the question is:

Why is it not working?

Why does the traditional method fail to help us?

Why can't we liberate ourselves going this way?

And also:

Is the traditional approach the only way to deal with PMO?

Answering those questions, surely, should be the first step of our walk together, the start line of our inquiry. Shouldn't it?

Brother, isn't it important for you to know why all your efforts to eliminate the addiction do not work?

You say you do see the importance?

For us, it is of vital importance. Not only because of the limitation in itself, but because finding the right answer to those questions reveals a lot about what we are as a human beings and clears the path for further inquiries, for deeper understanding of the human condition.

Our walk starts with a "**Why**".

However, let's not bother ourselves with theories and conclusions, let's just walk and see where it will lead us. Let's see those questions as an invitation to move together with great curiosity and genuine interest in understanding our problem.

Please see this: How we approach those questions is very important.

First of all, each one of us must understand clearly why we are asking them and you should not accept them just because this book is telling you they are important. But you have to see for yourself the importance of those questions and why it is imperative to find the answer.

That's why we insist on moving together. If you are merely following some words or someone else's philosophy, you will be left behind or worse you will be just imitating and will never know the joy of discovering something for yourself.

We are working as brothers with the same interest, the same drive and the same condition. That means we are inquiring, analyzing and exploring freely, diligently, without rushing or assuming anything, slowly, helping each other.

So as brothers, we ask you not to just accept what we say, but please take notes, write down somewhere what you think and all the ideas what we expose triggers in you.

Don't let it go, get yourself a journal and write it down. Be it small, crazy or insignificant, write it down. You will see for yourself how helpful it is.

Have your pen ready?

Awesome!

Let's dive in!

The Battle

"A broken mind..."

Have you ever seen a good car engineer repairing a motor?

Have you noticed how they intuitively know sometimes what problem the car has by simply hearing the sound it produces?

You know why they can do that?

It is because they know how a car works. They have studied in detail the internal operation of cars, their systems and accessories. And that knowledge gives them the ability to recognize and fix the issues of any car.

What about we should follow that same principle?

In order to discover why the traditional method does not work, we must first understand the essence of it, the idea behind it. And then, by having a good comprehension of it, we can see for ourselves where and why it fails.

If you agree, let's dig into that old way of dealing with the urges and the whole problem of addiction to PMO (pornography, masturbation and Orgasm).

Together we are going to dive deep into that system all of us have been following for years with the hope of producing that so desired transformation.

You see, when we follow the traditional approach, which is to fight and resist, we automatically create conflict within ourselves. A division between you and the thing you must resist, between **"You"** and PMO, between **"You"** and the addiction.

When you go that way, your mind is broken into two apparently separated pieces, and those two sides are going in opposite directions, they are in constant conflict, in constant war.

This is very clear and each one of us can see it in ourselves. You have certainly experience this everlasting friction going on in your mind, your body, your mood and your guts when you try not to relapse. This inner confusion you find yourself in after seeing some provocative pictures on Instagram, for example.

That is the battle between those two parts.

A violent confrontation between a "Fighter and his Opponent". Between the one resisting, struggling, fighting and the other one trying to express and impose itself.

This is the first obvious thing we encounter when we begin to question that movement which we all follow, the movement of resisting the urges.

We see a violent war, a movement of opposition and contradiction, a split of the mind in two opposite sides. One fighting, resisting and the other one receiving all the blame, being repressed.

"**You**" against "**That**".

"**You**" against "**PMO**".

"**You**" against the urges.

Now, let's scratch it a little more.

What it is we are trying to do by creating that division in our mind?

What is the aim?

You see, the idea behind this approach is to identify yourself with the part that suppresses and resists until you reach a point where the urges no longer show up. Isn't it?

You want to destroy the urges, to eliminate them completely from your life.

And to do that, in order to achieve that state of freedom, people have invented all the methods you certainly have tried or heard about. They are all over the internet.

If you go on google and search for: *"How to quit porn addiction"*, or *"How to stop masturbating"*, all kind of methods, a huge list of ways will be given to you as an answer to your **"How"**, as an answer to your desire to be free from that deep psychological pain you suffer.

And, when you really look at them and question what is being offered, when you gaze seriously into this gamma of procedures, methods, steps and systems over how to deal with the addiction, you soon find that they are all pointing to one single thing.

They all emit one single message, the exact same particular idea.

All the teachings say: **"*Fight, resist and control, one day you will be free!*"**

That's the message, isn't it?

Fight, be strong, use this method, apply that method and you will be free from the addiction!

And it sounds fairly logical.

After all, when you think about it, that's how we, as human beings, deal with anything that bothers us in life…

Conflict, violence and destruction!

And that's totally fine…

You see, we are not condemning or trying to influence anybody. That's not at all our intention. As we have said in the previous chapter, we don't bother with conclusions.

Our mutual and brotherly concern is to explore what we encounter, questioning and inquiring into what we see in order to understand why our efforts in that system do not bear fruits.

Are we together, brother?

Great! Let's keep moving.

So, the next thing we encounter when we question the movement is a certain hope, an expectation, the belief of reaching something at the **"end"**.

And because of that, we hold on to a streak, we count the days until we reach what we think is at the end of our struggles.

We suck the pain up when we relapse and get back on track. The battle must continue. And even though we relapse again and again, we still go after "It" hoping the urges will magically stop one day, hoping things will be better in the future.

In that sense, the essence of this traditional approach in dealing with the addiction is this:

"To divide our mind in two opposite fragments and to identify ourselves with that particular fragment fighting, trying to destroy the other one, believing

that when he achieves that goal, all his fantasies and expectations will be fulfilled."

That's the simplest way to put it. Please, feel free to analyze it yourself and to add the details you think we have left out.

This is the central idea behind all your fights and all your resistance in the journey, isn't it?

You move in that pattern, in that particular sense.

And, the sad truth is that we have been going that way for years. Some of us for three years, others for five years, and still others for a much longer time, struggling and hoping; Failure after failure, chasing that state at the "end" which will provide a sense of freedom.

But, at the end of the day, you are still burning with urges and suffering...

You have tried all the methods of the successful "warriors".

Time after time you have said to yourself: "***That's it, I won't fall back this time***". But the next thing you know is the urges taking over and forcing you to relapse.

Each one of us, we know that sad and depressing situation very well.

Now, if we can see this fact clearly, we must admit to ourselves that something is missing or malfunctioning.

Because, you see, for the vast majority of us, no matter how strong our determination seems to be, we cannot handle the urges when they show up and we end up giving in to them and failing to keep the streak.

Something is obviously not at its place!

What do you think it is, brother?

Having understood what the traditional approach, the way of the Fighter, is all about and seen clearly that it fails to help us, can you see where the malfunction in the system is?

We must find that out because, all of us, we have faith in that system. We have put all our hope for a change in that particular approach and we keep holding on to it even though, deep down, we feel great despair and misery.

So, let's find out together what the issue is.

The Fighter

"An unraveling rope…"

Quick question brother:

Why do you fight your urges to relapse in the first place?

See, we are not saying you should or should not fight, but we are simply asking why, why do we go on resisting? Why do we always feel the need to resist and to oppose ourselves to that thing which is present and factual in us?

Why are you trying to destroy your deep tendency to masturbate and watch porn?

Why among all the ways we could approach the issue, why do we <u>choose</u> to be its enemy?

That's a scary question, isn't it?

Who is the fighter? Who is fighting whom?

That's where the loophole of the system can be found.

When you observe yourself and the way you struggle with the addiction, you realize that the Fighter is not strong enough to defeat the part of you that wants to relapse. He may appear to have great energy and determination in the beginning, but your willpower lasts only for a couple of days or weeks and then weakens in down spiral till it crashes into a terrible fall.

That's our actual reality and we cannot close our eyes on it.

Seeing that fact, we understand that the movement or the tendency in us we identify as the **"Fighter"** is the defective component of the system. Clearly, it is where we are stuck. So, we must pursue our walk in this direction and look at the origin of the Fighter, his movements, what he is made of and why he cannot bring the liberation we want.

The Fighter is basically a movement of will; it is your willpower in action, going in a particular direction. Our observation has revealed how unstable it is and how it cannot sustain itself.

For some time, it seems powerful and in control of the urge but in the heat of the battle, it loses its power and leaves you alone, by yourself.

It's like hanging over a cliff, holding onto a slowly unraveling rope until you fall.

All of us, we know this very well.

After a relapse, we say to ourselves with frustration and determination:

- *"That was the last time I did it!"*
- *"It will be different from now on!"*
- *"Next time I won't fall!"*
- *"I will do everything to keep my streak!"*
- *"I have a goal"*.

Even though you know deep down this is a lie you are telling yourself, you keep it going because it comforts your self-image.

So, you do everything you can to maintain that rush of energy alive until the urge strikes and destroys it. Then goes the relapse and you recreate the same pattern.

When you identify yourself with the Fighter, you get caught in this pattern. Your hope and the relapses form a series of ups and downs with the Fighter, **"You"**, in between.

You alternate the relapses and the regains, the downs and the ups.

Of course, this pattern also shows how unstable and weak we become when we choose the path of resistance. We set ourselves for failure because the tool we are using is not fit for the battle.

We will see together in the next chapter why the Fighter is not the right instrument to obtain what you are looking for.

The Judge

"A reservoir of blame…"

You don't resist and fight yourself for no reason. The Fighter gets his energy somewhere; your willpower is motivated by something, obviously.

You are always acting and moving in a certain direction.

Because when you say ***"I must not masturbate"***, you are saying this for various reasons. Those reasons can be religious, medical, personal and so on.

All of those reasons are what fuel the Fighter; they are his origin, the motive behind your resistance. Therefore, if we want to understand why the Fighter is deficient, we have to look at this reservoir of motives where he is originated and where he receives his commands.

You fight, primarily, because you are desperate for a change, you want this thing to stop manifesting itself, to disappear; you want things to be different.

Why is it so?

You resist, you create an opposition, and you try to distance yourself from what is present and actual, It is clear.

But, why?

Why are you so desperate to be different? Why are you trying to negate, to tame or to alter what you actually are?

Isn't because you hate how you currently are?

Isn't it because you have labeled masturbation as something bad?

Isn't that labeling the central cause of this appalling inner battle?

You go on fighting and resisting because you believe the thing you are addicted to, to be an ugly and shameful practice, something you should not be doing under any circumstances, something highly prohibited. Don't you?

Why? Where does that belief come from?

Have you ever asked yourself why you think that way?

It is important to ask this question because, you know, science has discovered a variety of animals, other than humans, that masturbate. Our cousins, the primates for example, have a strong inclination for self-pleasure. Elephants, turtles, bats and even lizards also show the same tendency.

The only thing is:

For those creatures, it is not at all a big deal, just a natural and healthy practice.

Some of them do it after mating to protect themselves from infections transmitted sexually and others just for pleasure.

For us humans, it is seen as one of the vilest, most degrading and unhealthiest practices. That's the idea that we have inherited and we can feel the reality of it in ourselves, in our daily struggle, in the thoughts we have after a relapse, especially when we lose a long streak.

That idea is what we call "***The Judge***" in our community.

The Judge is seen as a great reservoir of blame, shame, condemnation, bad feelings and pure hatred directed toward the practice of Masturbation and Watching pornography, or PMO for short.

And it represents all the things, the methods, the sentiments, the emotions, the beliefs, the thoughts and the logics that keep the idea of opposition and resistance going.

The Judge is the hand that holds The Fighter; it is the actual fuel of your willpower. It is where we pick the impulse that makes us resist the urges and feel bad about ourselves when we fail to hold till the "end".

In more simple terms, The Judge is all the things we believe about the practice of PMO. The Judge acts and shows itself in our daily lives, when we have an urge, as The Fighter.

We then see together that the Judge is based on one single idea and that idea can hide itself behind many reasons; It can disguise itself in so many different ways. Some of them are obvious and some others pass totally unseen by most of us.

So, in our pursuit of understanding fully why the Traditional Approach fails to free billions of its adepts, all the brothers around the world and of previous generations who thought fighting and resisting would bring liberation from the addiction, we must explore the disguises of The Judge.

But before we go into such an arduous task, there is one thing to keep in mind... The expression of The Judge varies from one brother to another brother, which means it has a personal touch to it.

For sure, this is the same movement, similar in direction, but it is different in the ways of expression. The reasons that convinced you to strive for liberation are not always the same as those of another brother in the same struggle. It may be the same aspiration, the same movement of the Judge but not the same fuel. Do you see what we mean?

That's where your contribution is very important!

We suggest you to take note of the personal reasons you have for this aspiration.

Your personal reasons to fight the addiction can be described as your individual disguises of the Judge.

This process of bringing awareness in your own ideas is of vital importance because, after all, only you know yourself as deeply as you can be known and only you can understand why you are the way you are. Don't you?

We can help you ask yourself the right questions, we can point you toward the doors and we can assist you on a general scale but we can never personalize it for you, can we?

It is then down to the individual responsibility of each one of us.

With that clearly established, let's continue our mission!

Disguises

"Myths and beliefs…"

How do you know masturbation is wrong?

Please brother, we are not saying it is or it is not, we are simply asking how this label came to you. Who taught us to see masturbation as something we must be ashamed of?

We have seen the same practice in other creatures and for them there is no shame whatsoever but in our case, we run away from it, we cover it, we try to escape from it and we disguise those attempts of escape with reasons and motives.

"Masturbation is bad, don't do it" That's what they say and because they say that, we must follow it and beat ourselves up each time we do that "bad" thing.

But who are **"They"** who categorize masturbation as wrong?

Who is that supreme entity that dictates how you should feel about masturbation?

Who has decided to make it an evil and shameful practice rather than a natural act?

Who is it?

Society, isn't it?

All the reasons and the motives we have to activate the Fighter come from society or are derived in some way from it. All the judgements you pass on the practice of masturbation were picked up from what you have heard or been taught.

What a realization!

"The Judge is actually the voice of Society in our head, not ours."

What we refer to as **Society** is our parents, our doctors, our religious leaders, philosophy, social Medias, news, trends, the experiences, the reactions, the beliefs and all the sources where you get your conception of Life from.

The difference between the animals and us is that we are actively social creatures. We live together, we relate, we share our experiences, we can convince each other of our ideas and perspectives. Your social life is a share of the collective human interpretation of things.

Because we live in society and depend on it, we accept everything that goes with it. This is also the case with The Judge. All the reasons we have to keep the Judge moving were given to us, directly or unconsciously, since we were a little child by society.

Those reasons we have accepted from society become our motives, they become the things we strive for or we want to avoid.

Let's see together the common and most popular reasons the Judge holds on to, let's take a look at the disguises.

There is this belief that masturbation is bad for your health. We have all heard that excessive masturbation will lead to blindness or some vision disorders. There are also other medical claims such as:

- *Hairy palms*
- *Infertility*
- *Erectile dysfunction*
- *Hair lost*
- *Penis deformity*
- *Prostate cancer*
- *Mental disorders.*

And even though science has been able to show no evidence to verify those claims, they are still deeply anchored in the minds of most of us.

Apart from the medical disguises, religious leaders have been, for ages, telling us that masturbation is a sin and those who enjoy the practice will go to hell and suffer for eternity.

That's why you have the story of Onan in the Bible, where the term **"Onanism"** to refer to masturbation comes from.

You have the Paedagogus of Father Clement of Alexandria who depicts the practice as **"Wastage of divine seed"**.

You have the Panarion of Father Epiphanius of Salamis which describes it as **"Corruption"**.

And of course, you have modern catechism and the most popular religions of the world which label masturbation as an immoral and unnatural act.

Our families and friends, being part of society, repeat those same beliefs and have passed them on to us either by telling us directly or by making us feel guilty and ashamed for it. They keep the whole thing going as a tradition, as a code of conduct, as values.

Added to that all our personal and individual bad experiences derived from the practice and the realization that we cannot prevent ourselves from relapsing, we create this sense of negativity around masturbation and a huge reservoir of shame and blame you carry with you all the time.

This great reservoir held in place by the single original idea of masturbation being something fundamentally wrong, is what we call **"The Judge"**.

All of those medical, religious, philosophical beliefs and so on, depart from that single idea, from the Judge.

So, we have the central idea around which rotate all the different reasons that justify it and this justification acts through willpower as resistance, as conflict, as the will to fight, as opposition, as escape, as fear, as pressure, as this sense pf struggle, of hustle and through all the methods we use as a means to destroy the addiction.

The Judge, which is our movement of labelling the practice of masturbation as something wrong, is inciting us to create a battle within our own mind. That's how we have created the Fighter.

Brother, if we may, let us remind you that we are not rushing anything, we want to go as clear as possible, that's why we move slowly, with hesitation into this very complex exploration. We are digging into a system that has been in our minds for ages but which has failed to free us from our problem.

Our current concern is to find out why we are not able to get the results we desire following this traditional system.

By now, we believe, you have a clearer view and understanding of the Traditional Approach, the system that billions of brothers trust to relieve them from the grip of PMO.

The Traditional Approach, as we have discovered together, consists in accepting and following the negative voice of Society running all the time in your head, empowering you before and after a relapse to fight and resist what you consider to be your enemy.

In simpler terms, The Judge with many Disguises is sustaining all this violent conflict and inner struggle you experience.

That is clear enough, right?

Let's scratch a little more.

Expectations

"Don't be a fool..."

The Traditional Approach has evolved through time and with the invention of the Internet, it has exploded all over the place, becoming more and more subtle, disguising itself in even more subtle ways.

One of the most popular communities of modern society that perpetuate the Traditional Approach is the website or the movement known as: **"NoFap"**.

The name came from the American slang: "To fap" which means to masturbate and it has been all over the Internet since 2011.

The idea behind it is the same that has been around for generations:

To fight and resist the urges to masturbate.

The only difference is that you don't have to do it by yourself, you don't struggle alone in your little corner, you have thousands of guys who are "open" about it through forums, chats and more recently through videos. And those few who have been fighting and holding themselves for a long time (generally a year and above) are seen as teachers or gurus by sharing their achievements and the methods to get the same results.

Sounds effective, right?

 You see, this new generation of The Judge which refers to itself as the "NoFap Community" or just "NoFap" has created another set of Disguises for the Judge even more superficial than the previous one.

Before the explosion of the NoFap movement, we were avoiding and fighting masturbation because we thought it would bring harmful consequences, detrimental side-effects to our physical and spiritual health but nowadays, with the methods of the NoFap gurus, we are fighting and struggling to get rewards.

Do you see the evolution?

First, the Judge had only a negative set of disguises. Now, the Judge has invented another set of disguises, a positive one to add more strength to its self-justification and to give even more power to the actions of the Fighter.

As you probably well know, in the NoFap Community, there is the keeping of streaks.

You hold yourself, you fight, and you resist the urges to relapse until you reach a number of days which has been previously fixed as a goal or that somebody else has told you to strive for.

The most popular streak is the famous 90 days challenge.

You try not to watch any porn videos and not to touch yourself for 90 days. And you believe you will get something out of it. You think you will get attraction from girls, more confidence, charisma and all the good things those who have done it make you think you will get.

And you go day by day fighting, resisting the temptations, coping with the urges, repressing them, doing whatever you can not to fall back.

You do that because you are expecting what was promised to you.

And the funny thing is that you don't even know if what they have promised you is true or not. The only thing you know is that you must fight and resist and consequently, living in the constant fear and anxiety of failure.

You beat yourself up when you fail to keep the streak.

Whenever you feel the urge, you must apply the methods; torture yourself to barely make it to those famous 90 days.

You are addicted to the idea of NoFap.

You are so obsessed with your expectations. You are so desperate to achieve what was promised to you by those gurus and heroes of NoFap.

Your obsession is such that the number of days becomes more important than your transformation itself. And It's really crazy to see how some of us are so mad on this.

- *What will happen if I don't jerk off for 30 days?*
- *What will happen when I complete the 90 days monk mode challenge?*
- *When will my brain starts to rewire?*
- *When will I stop craving for porn videos?*

Just a bunch of hopes, expectations and promises!

We are so caught up in those expectations and speculations that most of us have become so vain, utterly unrealistic and very superficial.

You know, to say the truth, those things can be helpful if you know how to use them properly. They can keep you motivated to a certain extend but here we are asking if this is really your case.

"**You**", personally!

Do those promises really prevent you from relapsing over and over?

Did they magically make your last urge go away?

Or in the heat of your pressing and burning craving for porn and masturbation, all those promises, those methods and your expectations disappeared?

If they have helped you, feel free to keep following them. But if it is not your case, if you keep relapsing over and over despite you have watched thousands of videos on NoFap and read countless articles about it, then it is a clear indication that you should change your approach.

You are a fool if you keep betting on the same number when the horse is clearly not fit to win the game.

You are a fool if you keep using the same strategy and taking the same road when all you get is failure.

Your expectations, however strong and pleasurable they may sound, cannot save you from the urges. And that's exactly why you keep relapsing.

Don't be a fool, brother.

It is simply not working and those of us who are really serious about bringing a definitive change in our life, must admit it to ourselves.

And those of us who are not really serious about it can keep watching and enjoying their little memes…

Anyway, now, we are getting to the heart of the problem with the fighter and the reason why all our efforts to change do not bear fruit and why all this violence and pressure we put on ourselves is useless.

Can you see it?

Let's go into it together!

Head vs Heart

"Talk is cheap…"

As we have discovered, the Judge, which represents all the reasons why you are resisting the urges, all the motives you have to attempt the 90 days challenge and all the drive behind your need to fight your attachment to porn and masturbation, is disguising itself with both a negative and a positive sets of justification.

The first set of justification for all this self-inflicting torture is because we want to avoid the harmful consequences of masturbation.

You try to escape from the addiction maybe because you don't want to be blind or to lose your hair and get bald.

Maybe it is because you don't want your memory to be affected.

Perhaps your family or your faith taught you it is sinful and you will be punished for that on the judgment day.

Maybe you have read somewhere that excessive masturbation will prevent you from having children and you don't want that to happen.

Maybe it's because you don't want to lose your virility in the bed.

And you certainly don't want people to see your hairy palms.

See, we all have something we believe to be a harmful consequence of masturbation and we are fighting ourselves not to do it whenever we feel the urges coming.

Please, don't forget to write down in your personal journal the negative consequences you are personally trying to avoid when it comes to masturbation.

Now, the second set of justification for fighting your cravings for masturbation is to attain the promises and expectations.

We all want the satisfaction of having reached 90 days without touching ourselves. The pride there is in being a successful **"nofapper"**.

Maybe you try to destroy the addiction because you want more attraction from girls.

Perhaps you want to have more focus, more energy.

You want to increase your self-confidence.

Again, feel free to write down in your journal the gains you are looking for in this journey.

We are all looking to achieve the tempting results promised by the NoFap gurus and those who claim to have developed superpowers and incredible social abilities after quitting masturbation for a certain period of time.

Those two types of justification are what keep you fighting and struggling against your strong attachment to masturbation.

They are what is acting through you when you say: **"No! I won't relapse this time"** even though every cell in your body and every beat of your heart are moving in the sole direction of the relapse.

They are what makes you believe this time will be different even though deep down in your conscience you know falling back is the only outcome.

Time after time, relapses after relapses, day one after day one, you receive the obvious message that the Judge and the Fighter cannot prevent you from relapsing.

So, why is it so?

Why, despite you believe masturbation is bad and you clearly are against it, why can't you stop?

Why does the Judge/Fighter fail?

Did you see the reason?

The reason is clear and obvious brother.

All those things you believe about masturbation and fight yourself for are not your actual reality!

They are clearly operating in a dimension below or above your attachment to porn and masturbation and they have no effect on it.

Because, when you say: **"I will not do it again"**, it is coming right from a place of illusion. You are affirming something you know is not true. You are lying to yourself.

You know, there is a very "to-the-point" quote for that:

"Talk is cheap"

It's like when we say: **"Hell yeah! Tomorrow I will wake up at 6 AM to work out!"**

But will you actually get out of bed when the 6 AM alarm rings?

Most probably no.

The Judge and the fighter which is your actual instrument against PMO is just a bunch of ideas.

They don't really have a real meaning to you.

They are only in your head.

And not in your heart.

Take for instance when someone says: **"Please don't watch porn because there is sex trafficking in it. Little children are being abused because of pornography!"**

This information is very true.

But will that prevent you from actually having urges and watching porn videos?

Will that magically turn off your burning desire for those kinds of videos on the internet?

Even though it is a reality in the sad and brutal world of pornography that innocent people are being mistreated and abused, it means absolutely nothing to you!

You don't feel their pain.

You don't really care about that fragile little girl kidnapped from her parents, drugged and forced to do horrible and damaging things just to fulfill fantasies.

Some innocent people will never have a normal life, but that's not your problem.

You have no feeling of empathy for them whatsoever…

If it was the case, if you really knew and care just a little for those unheard victims, you would never open the incognito tab again. No doubt about it.

That may sound harsh but this is the plain-spoken reality and we are putting no makeup on it, dear friend.

Anyways, ideas, beliefs, logics, explanations, and all the things that form and sustain the Judge/Fighter, vanish when you are actually confronted with the urge.

They just disappear and leave you by yourself when you need them the most.

You can see it this way:

Let's say you have a group of friends with whom you often hang out, you guys drink together, laugh together and say you will always be there for each other in difficult times.

And, you trust them, you believe their words…

But imagine those guys you trust are never there for you when you truly need them.

None of them showed up when your grandfather died. They all disappeared the day you got beat up in the nightclub. Not a single one of them defended you the day you got arrested.

But yet, you still hang out with them...

Yet you still listen and believe their words.

Yet you still say: **"Oh, they didn't help me that time, but they will be there for me next time!"** Even though, countless times they have shown you their real faces.

Only a fool would do that, right?

Well, those who still hang onto the Judge, which is to fight the urges and resist themselves with the idea of avoiding bad consequences and attaining good qualities, are unconsciously doing the exact same thing.

They lie to themselves and say things they know they will not be able to respect.

They say they will not fall back into the sweetness of masturbation but quickly forget their decision in the next couple days.

Sound like someone you know?

Brother, we are not saying that to make you feel bad or to hurt your feelings but we want to make it obvious that the path we used to take is illusory and is not delivering the results we need.

We want to be clear on the fact that we are living an illusion and pretending to have some strength we know we lack.

We keep on repeating the same lies to ourselves day after day, relapses after relapses hoping somehow to generate a change, expecting things to magically be different one day.

We play this double game.

Now, the real question here is:

Why do we keep hanging onto the Judge/Fighter when clearly it is not helping?

Why do we keep condemning and fighting masturbation when we are secretly (or obviously) craving for it?

Why do you keep saying you want to destroy the part of you that enjoys watching porn videos and masturbate to them when every cell in your body is vibrating only for that?

And why do we, as society, feel the need to hate that part of us?

Why does society put a label on it?

Don't you want to find that out?

The Fear Of Masturbation

"Let's build a loving wall..."

Most of us are so embarrassed and feel so uncomfortable to talk about masturbation. It is one of the things in life everyone does but no one dare to talk about it.

And if you do talk about it, you will feel an atmosphere of awkwardness floating in the air.

Society has installed a heavy stigma around the act of masturbation.

With your share of this social conditioning, you fight your tendency to enjoy the practice. You repress your demands for it. You try to eliminate the urges either by convincing yourself they will bring some harmful physical, mental and spiritual consequences or by wanting some kind of future gains and achievements.

Clearly, we have something against it though we all enjoy it.

So why do we, as a society, hold that huge cloud of repression, guilt, shame and discomfort over the act of masturbation?

Why is masturbation such an evil thing?

Why is it that the very thing which provides you great pleasure is viewed as one of the most shameful acts you could possibly do?

Please, we are not hinting that you should indulge into unbridled masturbation, we are just asking ourselves, why is it that, despite we enjoy masturbation and all the pleasure, the sweetness, the bliss, the satisfaction that come with it, why despite this undeniable fact that we love it, why do we keep telling ourselves it is wrong?

Why do we play this double game?

Why this hypocrisy?

It is highly important to decode this as it is our life, our daily confusion. If you are really serious, you understand the necessity of asking _and_ answering such question.

Because, this hypocrisy is the very source of the harsh blame and hatred you put on yourself every single time you relapse.

So, why do you condemn your attachment to masturbation?

It is time for us to question this, even though it may be a little scary or uncomfortable to go into it and really touch the very bottom of it. It is time for you to see clearly where you have been standing all this time. It is time to look at your own confusing movement.

Let's approach it in a very simplistic way, brother.

Let's go back in history, when masturbation was practiced or discovered for the first time.

The idea with this approach is to get our mind around the thinking process behind this stigma placed over the practice.

Let's say, we are in the times of the first human social life form and we live in caves and have some kind of community. And you are the first man to discover the pleasure of masturbation.

We don't know exactly when the practice begun but let's assume it was around that time. The exact period doesn't matter.

Here you are one night, by yourself in your cave and you begin to pleasure yourself. You feel all the sweetness, tenderness, sensuality and ecstasy of the simple act of playing with your intimate organs.

You are excited, curious because it is a personal field you have never explored before.

And you enjoy it.

The moment you reach the climax of orgasm, you realize that sexuality is not just about reproduction or mating and you don't actually need a female to reach that state of bliss.

You're so excited!

Six months have passed and during that time you have being falling deeper and deeper into your secret passion day after day.

You no longer spend time with your community because, think about it, you have discovered a much more pleasurable, less stressful, less demanding way to spend your time. But you somehow still manage to stay around them.

One year after, you have noticeably changed. You begin to exclude yourself slowly from the others and surprisingly, you haven't mated with any female since then…

Three years have passed.

And one day, while chasing with your group, you feel that burning sensation in your belly. Suddenly you have this strong urge to withdraw yourself and have some personal joy.

Which you do…

You leave the others and go somewhere no one can see you to satisfy your pressing desire.

After you're done, you go back to them.

-*"**Where were you mate?**"* Someone asks

-*" **uhh... I had to go back looking for my weapons...**"*

You lie and hide your little secret.

This situation goes on for some time and you soon realize how addicted you have become to your own inclination and overall how it is affecting your relationship with your peers.

So, you try to stop, but in vain.

You are ashamed of it, of yourself.

And seeing how much control this thing has on you, you develop naturally a certain fear toward it.

That's the **fear of masturbation!**

You are afraid of the very thing that gives you the highest pleasure you currently know. Not that masturbation is the highest form of pleasure but right now, at this state of your life, it is.

You are afraid of it because it is going on without your consent. It leads you where you consciously don't want to go. And that's what the addiction means. You have become a slave to something you find great pleasure in.

And because of that fear, you have built this huge sphere of blame, of disgust, of shame, of guilt and of hatred around this little act which you cannot stop doing over and over.

You build a wall around it in order to protect yourself and all your efforts are only to strengthen this wall.

It is very important to see this: All your efforts are still in the realm of the addiction because it is a reaction to it, therefore part of it

One way to understand this fear of masturbation is this:

Take for instance the story of our caveman, let's imagine he has children, what do you think he will teach them about masturbation?

Won't he transfer to them this same fear he has of that which he finds uncontrollable, mysterious and shameful?

Out of his love for his little boy, won't he install in his little mind this protective wall of shame, blame and negativity?

It's obvious, right?

That's much more complex than that but we have promised you to keep it simple and direct. Feel free to meditate on this on your own.

So, the Judge/Fighter, which is the idea of declaring war to your attachment to PMO, which is a form of hypocrisy, which is a form of pretention, comes from this deep fear.

It is because society is afraid of the brutal possessive and tyrannical nature of the attachment to masturbation, they have tried to protect you from it by installing in your head all those beliefs and ridiculous claims around it.

As we have seen in previous chapters, this wall is made of all sorts of bricks!

False medical claims, absurd spiritual claims, all kind of things they can use to make you fear and run away from it. It doesn't matter if those claims are true or completely idiotic; they pour them right into your mind to sustain that wall of fear.

As we have also seen, this wall of fear is not only made of negative beliefs but is also composed by a set of positive claims, the pursue of rewards for avoiding or neglecting your strong tendency to PMO.

Again brother, we feel the need to remind you that we are not condoning the addiction or encouraging it but we are merely examining the problem with honest eyes, telling the things as they are, without fear or shame.

NoFap is part of that wall of fear...

By NoFap we mean the movement of applying methods, of following streaks, counting days of fighting yourself and resisting in order to achieve the promised state of freedom, in order to have gains, to have attraction from girls, to have social confidence, to be like to the gurus who taught you those techniques.

This movement is nothing more than another set of bricks of this great psychological wall of fear built around the act of watching adult videos and masturbating to them.

The Judge/Fighter combination which is the creepy voice of society, which is NoFap, which is your wanting to fight and destroy your attachment, is a movement of fear.

Do you see it?

As society, because we are so afraid of this uncontrollably and dangerously satisfying thing all of us do, that we decide to put a barricade tape around it, the same way we do with crime scenes.

That barricade tape, that protective wall, which is shame, guilt and violence, is born out of this deep fear.

"I enjoy it but it controls me. My enjoyment becomes my own trap and because I am afraid of not having control over it, I throw all my anger toward it. I try to run away from it and I get mad and frustrated everytime I fail to escape from it."

Brother, this is such a tremendous insight to have!

Because seeing that clearly helps you understand where all your efforts are coming from and why they have not been able to liberate you.

The Wheel: The Vicious Cycle

"A confusing pattern..."

Now that we have gone into the depth of the traditional approach and understood the reason why it doesn't help us, let's put it all together and see it for what it really is.

You have this tendency, this inclination, this constant need to watch porn videos and masturbate to them. And this tendency or attachment expresses itself in your body and your mind as the urges, the burning desire to fall into the sweetness and sensuality of your own sexual energy.

The moment you feel the urge, the moment something triggers it, you panic, you freak out because you are afraid of it.

And out of that fear, you create a resistance to the urge, you fight it, you try to eliminate it, which is the movement of the Jugde/Fighter, the idea of your sexual expression being something to be ashamed of, something impure and sinful you must destroy, something you will be socially and psychologically rewarded for getting rid of.

But this idea, which is the protective wall installed in your mind by society, is not strong enough to prevent your strong attachment from acting in the direction of the relapse, because after some times, this determination and this willpower weaken and become powerless against the enflamed desire to watch porn and masturbate.

After enough resistance, enough cold showers, enough pushups and applying all the promising NoFap techniques, after enough torture, you give up and fall into the temptation, which is the relapse, the doing of the very thing you swore you would never do again.

You see, this impotence against your own tendency leads to all kind of guilt, all kind of regrets but most importantly, it creates a deep sense of self-hatred and blame.

You said you would never do it again, but yet you went back to it. As a consequence, internally, you lose your self-confidence, your self-worth which helps you reinforce to yourself the idea of doing something fundamentally wrong.

Then, with those feelings, you say to yourself: ***"I hate this! Next time, I will not fall"***

This is the regain after a relapse.

You anticipate the next urge and fantasy on how you would not fall into the trap, on how strong you will be when it comes.

But when the urge comes again, guess what?

You do the same exact thing.

You repeat the same exact pattern.

So there is a repetition, a pattern and this pattern is a vicious cycle.

In our community, we identify this vicious circle as the **"Wheel"**. To us, this pattern, this vicious cycle is the real addiction.

The unconscious identification with this confusing pattern is the real problem and that's why the traditional approach sets us for failure when it comes to dealing with the attachment to pornography and masturbation.

In fact, this vicious cycle is something you go through in your daily life, everytime you have an urge and fight it. Your efforts are always within this circle.

All your judgments on your attachment to PMO, all your fears, your methods of escape, your guilt, shame, low self-esteem, expectations, rewards, streaks, counting the days, following NoFap methods, your relapses, the 5 seconds of orgasm, your regrets and frustrations, all of those things which constitute the movement of the addiction, which is our actual problem, are contained in this vicious cycle.

If you see this, you certainly understand what we mean when we say: **"The Wheel is the real addiction"**.

Therefore, being the center of the problem itself, this pattern must be studied with extreme care and diligence.

We will go into it together, as brothers.

You see, this turning wheel, which is the whole movement of the addiction, is composed by four distinct parts or moments.

They are the following:

1- The Urge
2- The Resistance
3- The Relapse
4- The Regain

It starts with having this uncontrollable desire to have the juicy and blissful experience of orgasm through watching porn videos and touching yourself, triggered by something.

Something triggers the memory of it and wakes the sensitivity of the body, the attention of the mind and the power of the feelings toward the experience.

This trigger can be anything.

It can be:

- *Merely seeing a female Instagram model while scrolling on social Medias*
- *The innocent act of watching a normal movie sex scene*
- *A picture in a "**Recovery group**"*
- *The name of a porn actress*
- *A wet dream.*

Something external awakes the hunger and demand for masturbation.

That's how the urge begins.

The moment you feel this thing in your body, the moment you get triggered, the Judge/Fighter automatically takes over and try to repress it, to avoid its movement. You label what you are feeling, this pressing urge, as an enemy, something you must get rid of and you apply NoFap methods on it or you simply try not to fall into its temptation.

But when we use the Judge/Fighter as a mean of stopping the addiction, we are creating more tension in ourselves. There is a tension building up till this resistance touches its peak and begins to weaken.

What is important to understand here is the fact that the Judge/Fighter tendency is also an urge!

Obviously, not the urge for masturbation but the urge to do what you think is its opposite, the urge to conform to the idea put in your head by society about masturbation.

The **"urge to fight the urge"** in order to be free, to be socially normal, to avoid bad spiritual and medical consequences.

Instead of stopping the addiction, this urge to fight, which is the essence of the Judge/Fighter, is adding even more tension to the wheel, adding even more power to the vicious cycle and thus bolding the addiction even more.

This is obvious because, after all, it is a reaction to the urge. Isn't it?

You are fighting an urge with another urge and you think by doing so you will be free.

This illusion of resistance may go on for a while until it attains its climax, then it will begin to lose power and direct itself toward the relapse.

But, you generally hold on to it.

You watch one video, two, three...You edge, but you still think you will not fall.

This little game can last for days and even weeks.

And finally, when you cannot hold it no more, you give up.

You relapse, you let go, which means you realize how powerless you are against your own attachment to porn and masturbation. The reality of the vicious cycle burns the illusion of the wall, it kills your pretention to freedom, it destroys your fake determination.

And when you see this, when you realize how powerless you are, what do you normally do?

You go into the state of despair and regret...

For a while, you will feel hopeless, worthless, impure, guilty and the sense of having lost the greatest battle of your life, won't you?

As we are seeing, all this is also part of the vicious cycle as it reinforces the Judge/Fighter.

They go together because in the next stage of the wheel, which is the regain, the Judge/Fighter will take over again as a reaction to the relapse, as frustration.

During that time, the Judge/Fighter anticipates the next trigger/urge and says: ***"It will be different next time, I will not fall again!"***

But when the urge comes back, it repeats the same pattern.

Over and over again...

This means that the cycle is sustained by your constant reactions to your attachment.

You react to the urge as the resistance and appliance of methods. You react to the relapse as the guilt, shame and the regain.

Those reactions are the compulsive movement of the Judge/Fighter, the urge to oppose to what you are so afraid of.

It's like when you are in a room with something you are afraid of, say cats, you react to every little movement they make, don't you?

You interpret every gesture as a threat.

That's the relation of the Judge/Fighter to the Urge/attachment, a movement of compulsive reactions.

So you have:

a) The urge triggered by something you associate with sexual pleasure,

b) Then you react to the urge as resistance, which is the idea of fighting and opposing yourself to something bad, wrong and sinful,

c) Then the relapse takes place and you react to that relapse as despair, sadness and frustration.

d) And, out of that frustration, you promise yourself to do better next time, but this is a big lie because you will repeat the same pattern again.

That's the wheel, the vicious cycle in which we are caught!

Each part of the wheel is a compulsive reaction, something happening unconsciously to your body and your mind.

The urge is a compulsive reaction to the trigger; the resistance is a compulsive reaction to the desire to watch porn and masturbate; the relapse is a compulsive reaction to the urge, guilt, shame and the regain is a compulsive reaction to the relapse.

We are caught in a series of compulsive reactions.

All those things seem to happen to you without your conscious contribution because you can't really prevent yourself from acting through those four specific movements.

Therefore, the addiction is not just the act of watching porn and masturbating to them but the addiction actually means the whole movement of this series of compulsive reactions!

Do you see this?

We are addicted to fighting the urges, which is the movement of NoFap, the Judge/Fighter combination.

We are addicted to the sweetness, the pleasure, the ecstasy of those five to ten seconds of orgasm, which is the relapse.

We are addicted to the guilt, the shame, the psychological self-punishment for having done something wrong.

We are also addicted to this feeling of anticipation, the pretention of being strong, which is the regain.

The addiction is all that!

The real issue is our identification with that turning wheel, our reactions in it, our pretentions, our little pleasures found in it, our ideas of freedom which are just reactions to it, that's the real addiction.

Unless this turning wheel stops or unless your actions become free from its compulsive movements, there can be no real freedom.

But, is that even possible?

Is it possible for us, each one of the millions of brothers around the world, after all those years moving through this wheel, identifying ourselves with this confusing pattern, after all those years caught in it, is it possible to be completely free from it, which is a total and lasting transformation?

Is that possible??

The Alternative Way

"Burn the lies..."

We started our brotherly journey together by asking ourselves why all our efforts to be free from this burden of attachment to pornography and masturbation do not work. Why, despite fighting and resisting relapses after relapses, why do we keep having our hands in our pants and our minds constantly searching for the pleasure of porn and masturbation.

To find an answer, we have been observing and examining together the way we traditionally approach our problem and unravel the reasons why it does not work.

We have discovered that the traditional approach is a movement of fear, which instead of liberating us, has enlarged the addiction furthermore, creating this confusing vicious cycle of the urge, resistance to the urge, relapse and regain from the relapse. It has created nothing more than a series of unconscious compulsive reactions.

One of the reasons why the traditional approach, which is NoFap, which is the Judge/Fighter movement, fails is because it is just a reaction coming from a place of fear and incapacity to come to terms with this burning desire we have to constantly enjoy our sexual expression.

Another important reason is the fact that it has become part of the attachment itself, adding more tension and power to the movement of the vicious cycle.

Seeing this situation, which is our daily life, our actual and factual state, seeing this clearly, we are then asking ourselves another very important question:

"Is it possible to break this confusing pattern and move in a totally new direction, outside of the wheel?"

Is it possible for our mind, finding itself comfortable and safe within this circle, to decide to step out of it?

You see, brother, this question is not about asking for a method or a technique to be free, but it's a challenge, not something you borrow from someone else, but a vital quest you, yourself, are going through.

You understand what this means?

Do you see the implication of turning your back to the traditional approach and thus the wheel?

It means that you have to stop looking for freedom as the outcome of compulsive reactions.

It means you have to turn your back on the idea of fighting the urges because the **"urge to fight the urge"** is a compulsive reaction. Compulsive reactions add more tensions and frustrations to the vicious cycle and therefore sustain it.

It means you have to turn your back on the whole culture of NoFap.

It means you have to negate the idea that someone or some method will magically make the addiction go away and you will never have urges again.

It means to stop counting the days, to stop going after superficial gains, to stop going after imaginary state of freedom.

It means to never listen to the voice of society in your head telling you: **"The urges are bad, masturbation is evil and sinful, it is dangerous for your health and your spirit"**.

This has to stop because those beliefs are sustaining the vicious cycle.

Moving outside the wheel or breaking the confusing pattern means to stand on your own!

To take 100% responsibility for your actions, to find out for yourself if there is a way to handle this urgent problem you are facing in your life, without being afraid of it because fear sustains the addiction.

Brother, aren't you tired of failing over and over?

Don't you have enough of this feeling of frustration, of being powerless against your own tendency?

Aren't you tired of living your life by default?

Aren't you tired of giving all your efforts, all your energy to only 5 to 10 seconds of pleasure?

Does the fact that you suffer with this thing every night mean nothing to you?

How do you feel, brother?

Don't you have in your heart this flame? Don't you want to finish with that burden for good??

Don't you want to live in a totally different way, a way without dependency, without compulsion and therefore with no pain and regrets?

Is fighting your urges to watch porn and masturbate the reason why you are alive??

How are you feeling now?

Do you feel it??

<u>THIS</u> is the beginning of freedom!

To be genuinely revolted, to have the sincere and serious feeling of the need for a change, on your own term, not borrowed from someone else, not even from us through this book.

To see for yourself the necessity for a deep transformation, not to just say it and follow some methods given to you by someone who say they know how to free you, but to let this frustration, this pain you have, to let it speak for itself.

If something true and lasting will come, it has to spring from that frustration, the same way a slave uses his pain to break his chain, the same way oppressed people set themselves free from tyrants.

Our actions must be true and free; they should not be derived from the Judge/Fighter and should not be corrupted by any method, which is just a form of fear in this case.

This situation of fear, of pain, of shame, of compulsiveness, of self-hatred, of inner confusion, of self-doubt, of self-slavery is your life, dude!

This is your daily experience, something only you can feel the way you feel it.

For that specific reason, only YOU can do something about it, no one on earth can teach you how to deal with it, nobody can do it for you.

It is your responsibility.

Taking 100% responsibility for your situation is the alternative way and this is the beginning of freedom!

To be free to inquiry for yourself with confidence and great curiosity, without external intervention or validation because external intervention creates conflict within you and produces undesired effects like guilt, shame and self-hatred.

And, you know, when you think about it, that's the real meaning of the word: "Responsibility".

It's interesting because for most of us, the word responsibility usually means to take blame for something not going well, to be guilty of something.

But when you do look at the word, it has nothing to do with blame, shame or guilt, on the contrary, it points to something far greater!

Respons-ibility is actually the ability to respond.

Your ability to respond, your ability to do what is needed, when it is needed and where it is needed. And, in that sense, responsibility is the essence of intelligence itself.

It is your intelligence acting when you are faced with a challenge, with a problem or an issue.

Here we have the greatest issue in our lives, the most significant challenge in our lives; we are slaves to our own vicious cycle, our own tendencies, our own urges and you need to respond, not reacting compulsively to it out of fear, but to use your intelligence.

See, reacting is one thing and responding consciously is a totally different thing. Reacting is unconsciousness but responding is a conscious action, a movement based on responsibility, on truth and intelligence.

If you really want to stop having this feeling of worthlessness, this psychological pain of guilt, of shame and low self-esteem, you need to assume total responsibility for the condition in which you find yourself.

It is your concern to find out what is happening to you, it is your job to understand it and it is your ability to respond with great intelligence to it.

Only you can do that.

Look brother, nobody can tell you how your hands feel, only you can have this experience.
Nobody can tell you how your breathe feels to you, only you can know that.
Nobody taught you how to derive pleasure from masturbation, you learned it by yourself.

Though the experience may have come to you through someone else, the feeling of it, the enjoyment of it, and the attachment to it were discovered personally, on your own.

You have put yourself into this hole and taking full responsibility is to know for a fact that no one but you yourself can take you out of it.

Any attempt of external help is doing nothing more than digging the hole even further.

Any judgment, any methods, any ideas picked up from someone else will do nothing more than creating more confusion, more conflict and therefore more pain.

You are on your own.

Responsibility also means to stop identifying yourself with the opposite of the addiction, to stop the pretention.

To be brutally honest with yourself.

To stop living in the illusion of not wanting to feel the pleasure of PMO, to stop pretending you hate it.

Let's be clear here, we are not saying you should keep masturbating and fill your mind with those videos, we are saying to stop lying to yourself.

Stop pretending to negate it.

Responsibility is to look at it exactly as it is, without makeup, without a distorted screen, to dive deep into the ocean of truth with oneself.

And understanding this fact is like planting a seed, you become a seed ready to grow but which knows its current state.

There must be no illusion, all the traps of the Judge/Fighter, all the deceptions of the Wheel to sustain itself must be wiped out.

If you see the necessity of such a drastic action, we wonder how you feel right now in relation to the addiction.

Now that we have gone into the core of the problem and understood the whole movement of it, the four distinct parts of it, how do you feel brother?

One day, you realized how addicted you are to PMO, you realized you cannot stop it from controlling your mind, your body and your actions.

It was very scary at the moment, you were afraid.

And because of that fear, you have adopted the traditional approach, which is NoFap, with the hope of getting rid of that problem. You started using the Judge/Fighter as a tool to transform yourself. But instead of helping you, it has added more psychological pain to that fear you had in the beginning by creating the Wheel, the vicious cycle.

Making you struggle relapse after relapse, urge after urge with the hope of attaining a state of freedom that has never come.

Luckily, through our conversations and inquiry, you have realized what was happening to you, you have become aware, not only of how useless and deceptive is the tool you were using to deal with the addiction, but most importantly why it can never bring the freedom it promises.

You have discovered it for yourself, you have seen the truth of it and you have decided to throw the useless tool away.

Now, how do you feel?

Don't you feel a certain relief?

Don't you feel free and more conscious?

It feels like a blue and clear sky after a stormy rain. Doesn't it?

Don't you feel like you have more energy, more drive?

It is so because your focus is more organized.

Your energy is no longer dissipating itself all over the place into illusions but is relatively stable.

Do you feel that?

You are no longer burdened with streaks, with running after gains, no longer confined into the compulsion of beating yourself up when the urge is present; no longer burdened with the Judge/Fighter and all his fears.

THAT, dear brother, is the magnificent power of responsibility!

Now that you have stopped following someone else methods, now that you have stopped neglecting to somebody else the work only you can do, you take your own responsibility.

That doesn't mean you become egocentric and vain, on the contrary, it means you have become a source of freedom, not a stuck rock only receiving help from outside but an active and independent force, which is, by the way, the real meaning of **"Self-help"**.

It is on you to deal with what is happening to you, you don't burden others with your problems, you don't depend on any method, any technique, any streak, and your freedom is intrinsic.

It is a perfume which accompanies you on every step you take.

And with that total responsibility, you have the power to inquiry into yourself and see for yourself what must be done and how to create another kind of life for yourself.

It is all on you!

What Is The Urge?

"Flow of creation..."

If there is one thing the study of the traditional approach and the wheel has shown us, it is the fact that we are very afraid to address the real issue, the fact that we neglect our responsibility to external forces.

It has shown us the real issue: **Fear**.

But, what it is we are so afraid of?

What it is we are endlessly running away from, constantly trying to resist, always trying to escape from?

What is that thing we enjoy so much but yet we are so ashamed of?

Brother, what does it mean to have an urge?

What is the meaning of this addiction, of your current psychological condition?

Who/what is that enemy you try to destroy?

Have you ever taken your time to quietly and seriously examine yourself this way?

Have you ever put away your fear of it, your judgements of it, your ideas of it, you willingness to change it, have you ever put aside all that and look at yourself exactly as you are?

With the eyes of honesty and humility in order to learn and understand what is happening inside our addicted mind.

That's real responsibility!

So, what is that thing you are so powerless against?

What is the urge and where does it come from?

When you observe it, you will see that it manifests itself in the body as this internal impulse, this ultra-sensibility you feel in the lower part of the body.

It manifests itself in the mind as the recalling of previous masturbation sessions, previous pleasure, previous orgasm and the anticipation of those 5 seconds blissful state.

We usually fight those manifestations when we see them in ourselves; and somehow we manage to view them as things *happening* to us.

But are they different from us?

Is the urge something separated from you? Or is it 100% your making?

Is there an external force pushing you toward that?

Or is it an internal demand?

You see, we cannot divide ourselves from the movement of the urges for we are their source.

The urge is obviously not an autonomous creation, it must be something we, ourselves we are doing. Isn't it?

The only thing is that we are not aware or conscious of how we create them...

Or we don't want to accept this fact.

The entity creating the urge is that same entity pretending to destroy it, therefore he runs in circles, chasing his own shadow, pursuing his own tail.

Taking responsibility for the urge, for the addiction, puts you in front of this crude truth, doesn't it?

The urge is your creation, your unconscious action.

When you feel the strong need to watch pornography and masturbate, it is not something you can run away from or apply method on or ask for external help for, it is an internal action, a fire you yourself have started inside of yourself.

No external water or sand can stop it, only you, the fire itself, can do something about itself.

Please brother, do see this!

This thing is your making, it is your life!

It is not an external, mysterious or evil thing imposed to you by some hidden demonic force. It is your own creation, isn't it?

So, why are you creating those urges?

Why are you constantly using your energy to create this hyper sensuality, this anticipation for orgasm?

Always remember, we are not condemning or encouraging it, we are just examining it. If you take position against or for it, you are still caught in the movement of the Judge/Fighter.

But rather, observe it, look at it, see it for what it is!

What is that uncontrollable thing?

Let's approach it as simply as possible.

For most of us, it starts with the need to watch porn videos or to get involve with something pornographic. But when you look very closely, you will see that porn is not the movement, but just a help for the movement.

You use porn as a mean to reach where you want to get, but porn in itself is not the "Thing", it is not what this impulse is all about.

Porn excites you, sets the mood, prepares you for what is about to happen.

You know, porn in itself doesn't happen on the screen, it happens in your mind, It is nothing more than the association of the representation you see on the screen with your sexual energy.

Come on! What we see on the screen or in the magazine has no real importance if no one consumes them. It is us who give life to them; it is us who use them as triggers.

Adding to that the fact that some of us don't even watch porn but still we are addicted to masturbation.

So, if porn is not the thing you are after but just a help to get it, then what do you want?

Keep it simple.

What it is you are looking for by expressing yourself through the urges and the act of watching porn videos?

Is it this deep sense of timeless enjoyment?

Could that be the reason why you find yourself on the verge of the relapse, ready to jump at any moment?

Safe and easy pleasure.

There is great pleasure and excitement in touching the most sensible part of your body.

There is a sense of **"beingness"**, a sense of existence, a feeling of presence in giving yourself totally to that act, isn't there?

There is this pleasure of being aligned with the movement of this timeless energy when you stop thinking and dive in the sea of the senses.

When you are in this state of excitement, you become extremely focused, responding to the slightest motion of blood in your body.

The world and all its problems disappear. Time has stopped.

You disappear.

There is only this blissful, ecstatic, unexplainable movement of the senses, the pleasurable memories, and the sense of reaching climax.

When you explode into orgasm, it's so refreshing, so rewarding, there is this great silence, a sense of cooling down after achieving a great prowess. Isn't there?

Everything you are, your body, your mind, your blood, your energy, everything, for a brief moment was in perfect synchronicity with the flow of life and you have abandoned yourself totally to that movement.

For your body, it was serving the highest purpose, which is to reproduce itself through the act of sexuality.

For your mind, it was serving the highest purpose, which is creation itself, the pleasure of creating with the sexual energy, the pleasure of putting aside the little "me" with its problems and flowing with the natural sexual force to create, to give life.

The pleasure of self-abandonment and total flow with creation.

The rewarding satisfaction of having given all you got to something. You can call it **"Dopamine"** or whatever you like, let's not get too scientific about it. Keep it simple.

Could that be the meaning of your attachment to PMO?

Please brother, don't just accept what we say, find out for yourself. It's an invitation to look for yourself. We have nothing to teach you, it's all your responsibility.

So, constantly looking for this easy and safe satisfaction, is that the reason why you are so attached to porn and masturbation?

Is that the meaning of the urges?

The Sexual Energy.

"The Creator's hand…"

When you think about it, it is weird…

We wouldn't be here, talking to each other and having this magnificent experience called **"Life"** without this mysterious force, without this impulse which allowed your parents to have you.

In fact, it is the origin of your family.

This is the origin of society itself.

Without this creative force/energy with which you are playing, from which you are deriving great pleasure and which you are throwing away so easily, we wouldn't exist.

Without this act, it would have been impossible to have seven billion people on this planet.

Shouldn't that power be something sacred?

Sacred, not in the religious sense, not in the way they have made us so scared of it and created all kind of stupidity around it.

But sacred in the sense of it being something highly precious, extremely valuable, more precious than any metal, any amount of money, more valuable than anything you can think of.

Something you should be very careful with, something you should preserve, something you should understand, something you should give your attention and diligence.

The source of your life... Not something you throw away in five minutes (or less).

Not something you waste on an illusory representation you see in a video but something you approach with great respect.

The basis of your existence... This is what sustains and continues life on this planet.

Not only did you come from this powerful energy, but you are also part of it, you can activate it and use it whenever you want.

In fact, your addiction means that you are using this powerful force unconsciously, so unconsciously that it seems like It IS using you.

See, there is nothing wrong with you, nothing wrong with being sexual.

Sexuality is a normal and natural expression of life. It is your capacity to reproduce yourself, to be part of the act of perpetuation of the human race.

It is important to understand this because most of us who find ourselves addicted to porn and masturbation, like to think there is a problem with us. We like to think we are defective.

No, you are not, brother!

Misusing a knife does not mean the knife is an evil instrument. The scalpel in the hands of a thief kills, but in the hands of a surgeon, it saves life.

In fact, it is not even about being good or bad; it's more about being conscious, self-conscious to be exact, which is the essence of responsibility.

Being sexual in itself is not the problem. What is blocking you right now is your level of consciousness and use of the sexual energy.

Look brother, what does sexuality mean to you?

Don't you have a highly conditioned vision and perception of your sexual energy?

For most of us who are addicted to porn and masturbation, the only touch we have of this energy is the excitement we get from porn or from our fantasies, our mental pictures and our distorted representation of the sexual intercourse.

Currently, sexuality means the sensation you get from touching yourself. It means the pleasure you get in ejaculation, in orgasm. Doesn't it?

And because of that, we also have to include into our experience of sexuality the heavy load of self-blame, of guilt and shame we carry after a relapse.

Sex has become the addiction itself.

Your experience of sex is within the field of the vicious cycle and sexuality for you is the wheel. The creative energy which allows all this to be possible is caught in this loop and you have never experienced anything outside of it.

You as the author of this force even though you are stuck into this constant circular motion of urge, resistance, relapse and regain.

Your energy is used to this pattern and it is constantly sustaining and protecting it because that's the only satisfactory expression it knows.

Do you see that?

It has become so comfortable within this loop that it is afraid to express itself in other ways.

It keeps creating excuses, false claims, all kind of illusions just to stay within its own limited and safe cocoon.

You, as this powerful and infinite creative force, choose to be this small, this limited, and so insignificant in your life on this planet.

Yes, it is a choice... but an unconscious one.

You choose to stay under the table and eat the little pieces of food that fall from the great banquet because you are so afraid of losing your little comfort, your little safety.

How come this magnificent creative power, which you are, which can create another human being, which can create an exquisite piece of art as the compositions of Beethoven, which can express itself through the Genius of Leonardo Da Vinci, of Nicholas Telsa, of Albert Einstein, of Alexander The Great and all the brilliant minds who have marked and inspired humanity, how come this vast reservoir of infinite creativity has become something so small, so repetitive and unconscious?

That's the same creative energy!

On a grossly physical level, it can produce semen and spermatozoids to create another human being. But on other higher levels it can produce so much more…

How come this energy which can create heroes, saints and avatars has become that "thing" which you waste and suffer?

How did that happen?

You know, seeing how limited this infinite creative energy has become, people started to talk about something called: **"Sexual Transmutation or Sublimation"**.

A term referring to the act of canalizing this creative force which expresses itself through the sexual movement to a higher expression of creativity such as social success, inventions, arts, spirituality and all the infinite possibilities one can access.

You are encouraged to move yourself from this current low expression to your highest possible manifestation.

This is a noble quest, but unless you understand the limitation and become totally aware of the deceptions you create for yourself to keep it going, unless you see clearly the traps you put in your own way in order to stay within this limitation, freedom or "higher expression" will always be a faraway dream.

Not only that, if you try to bring about that transmutation through suppression and resistance, you will be hurting yourself or worse the repressed desires will express themselves in other ways.

You see, the energy we express through sexuality is such an intrepid force!

You have certainly noticed how focused and concentrated you suddenly become the moment you have an urge.

How fearless, how sensitive, how alert and purposeful you become when you have to watch that video!

How it can't wait, how pressing, burning, explosive, insistent, persistent, strong and violent it gets when you have to do it! Nothing can stop you!

Brother, THIS is your power!

Imagine for a moment if you could put all that focus, that concentration, fearlessness and excitement into creating the kind of life you want, into achieving your most cherished dream...

Imagine how unstoppable you would be if all that count for you, right now, was to get those six figures mark in your bank account by the end of next year the same way all that count for you is to feel the ecstasy of orgasm when you have an urge...

Imagine if only one drop of this piercing, laser-focus and purposeful energy was directed toward what you most desire to achieve in your life...

Imagine if you could take it out of its current vicious cycle and give it its true meaning...

Imagine how powerful you would be!

But, for that to happen, this powerful life force must first become totally aware of itself, of its current limitation and only then with its own understanding can it effortlessly rise to higher realms, to higher expressions. Otherwise, it will create more harm to itself than good.

Total Freedom.

"Rise up..."

It has been our wish throughout this little guide to help you dive into the vast ocean of freedom.

Freedom, not only from the fear of the urges, not only from the fear of the relapses and their heavy psychological consequences, but most importantly freedom from the illusions of the Judge/Fighter.

Freedom from the need to neglect your responsibility to someone else.

Freedom from laziness, which means, to find the necessary energy to address the issue, by yourself.

Freedom from the idea of the urges being something external or mysterious, some kind of monster.

Throughout our journey together, as brothers, with this sense of freedom we looked at ourselves exactly as we are without shame, without any disgust or blame.

With this sense of freedom, we have been exploring quietly, hesitantly, with great concern and seriousness, the nature of our problem.

We have been free to go into it together, without any method, any technique, any teacher, any external guidance, without any so-called expert participation.

Free from the idea of freedom itself being something to achieve or something in the future. Free to look, to observe, to learn and understand yourself exactly as you are.

The sense of total freedom which comes not because you fight and create violence by imposing a certain discipline and order upon yourself, but this vitality, this clarity, this boost of energy and responsibility one naturally develops through self-education.

Our use of that word **"Freedom"** can be understood through the relation of darkness to light and the relation of ignorance to knowledge.

You see, darkness is **"what is"** when there is no light, the inexistence of light, therefore the only way to dispel darkness is with the presence of light. The moment you have one, the other is not.

The same goes for ignorance; it can only be shattered with the power of knowledge.

Light and Knowledge, which are the freedom to act, to create and express yourself, come into being only when you become really conscious of Darkness and Ignorance. Not to be afraid of them, not to react compulsively to them, but to truly understand them, to see their limitation and the principles hidden behind them.

That understanding is clarity, is the light itself!

It is like the rising sun springing naturally out of the dark night.

The moment you really feel the limitation and get a true sense of your potential, the revolution has already begun.

The same way the slow revolution of the planet lets us see the bright sun everyday, your revolution, which is self-consciousness and understanding, which is what we have been working on throughout this book, has to give birth to your total freedom!

It can't be otherwise!

Now dear brother, how do you feel?

Is there any addiction?

Is there any attachment?

Do you still want to keep moving into this limited vicious cycle in which you have a false sense of joy?

Or do you see exactly what it means to be part of this sacred elixir of life?

Your creativity, your genius, which is the essence of your life, can no longer be kept enslaved in the lamp and nor does it want to stay in. You feel it, don't you?

It wants to stop being mediocre, repetitive, misunderstood and misused. It wants to be expressed in its fullest possibility.

You are capable of so much more than using your energy to sustain illusions. You are not just an unconscious entity porn directors feed with fantasies in order to make money. You are not a lost empty boat being swept away by the waves of urges and relapses.

Surely, you are much more than that, aren't you?

It's time to rise!

Rise up, brother!

Now that you have withdrawn yourself from your own limitation and fears, are you ready to let us, the rest of world, see who you truly are?

Are you ready to show us your unique expression of this infinite power?

Are you ready to be the next Elon Musk?

Maybe someone far greater than Nelson Mandela, than Eckhart Tolle or Usain Bolt... Who knows?

Show us who you are!

Your share of this precious life force is unique and that's what makes you **"You"**.

We hope this guide has been able to open your eyes to how awesome each one of us is and how great we are destined to be!

Thank you for your seriousness and commitment to this.

And please remember:

You are not a mistake. You are a precious seed full of great potential and God knows how we can't wait to see what you will express in the world.

"May you fly like the majestic eagle over clouds and mountains"

With love,
Your brothers.

Break Those Chains.